Sample Meal Plan:
Menu For Diabetes And Muscle Atrophy Patients

Crystal Reed

Table of content

Chapter 1

What is the connection between diabetes and muscular atrophy?

Diabetes is a chronic illness that develops either when the pancreas does not create enough insulin or when the body is unable to use the insulin that is produced. A hormone called insulin controls blood sugar. Uncontrolled diabetes often results in hyperglycemia, also known as high blood glucose or raised blood sugar, which over time causes substantial harm to many different bodily systems, including the neurons and blood vessels.

Diabetes type 2
The body's inefficient utilisation of insulin leads to type 2 diabetes, also known as non-insulin-dependent or adult-onset.

Type 2 diabetes is characterised by improper insulin use by the body. And although some individuals can regulate their blood glucose (blood sugar) levels with good nutrition and exercise, others may need medication or insulin to do so. Whatever the case, you have all you need to combat it.

Diabetes Type 1
Diabetes type 1 (formerly known as insulin-dependent, juvenile, or childhood-onset) is characterised by inadequate insulin production and needs daily insulin therapy.

While it may manifest at any age, type 1 diabetes mainly affects children and young people. Type 1 diabetes may be more likely to develop if you have a parent or sibling who has the condition. Around 5% of diabetics in the US have type 1.

Several factors lead to type 1 and type 2 diabetes: Since the body's immune system destroys the insulin-producing islet cells in the pancreas, type 1 diabetes results in the pancreas not producing insulin. With type 2 diabetes, the pancreas produces less insulin than it once did, and your body develops an insulin resistance.

pregnancy-related diabetes
Gestational diabetes is hyperglycemia, which occurs when blood glucose levels are above normal but below those that are indicative of diabetes. Pregnancy is when gestational diabetes manifests.

Malnutrition, advanced age, heredity, inactivity, and certain medical disorders may all contribute to muscle atrophy. When you don't utilise your muscles sufficiently, you might have disuse (physiologic) atrophy. Nerve disorders or illnesses may cause neurogenic atrophy.

a kind of elevated blood sugar that affects pregnant women.

Individuals who have gestational diabetes are more likely to eventually acquire type 2 diabetes.

During extended inactivity, muscles might atrophy. The body will gradually break down unused muscles in order to preserve energy.

If a person is immobilised while recovering from an illness or accident, muscle atrophy from inactivity may develop. This kind of muscular atrophy may be reversed by engaging in regular exercise and physical treatment.

Muscle atrophy may be treated with specific lifestyle modifications, physical treatment, or even surgery.

What signs or symptoms may someone have diabetes?

Diabetes signs and symptoms include: heightened thirst and urination

increased hunger and exhaustion

eyesight that is hazy

tingling or numbness in the hands or feet.

unhealed wounds

Unaccounted-for weight loss

Type 1 diabetes symptoms might appear within a few weeks. Type 2 diabetes symptoms often appear gradually over a number of years and might be so subtle that you might not even notice them. Many patients with type 2 diabetes don't exhibit any symptoms. Some individuals are unaware they have the condition until they have diabetes-related health issues, such impaired vision or heart issues.

Signs of muscular atrophy
If any of the following applies to you:

Your arms or legs are notably shorter on one side.

One of your limbs has a noticeable weakness.

You haven't engaged in any physical activity in a very long time.

If you think you could have muscle atrophy or if you are unable to move properly, call your doctor to get a full medical checkup. There might be a medical ailment you don't know about that has to be treated.

Additional factors that contribute to muscular atrophy include:

prolonged inactivity

burn injuries, such as a ruptured rotator cuff or fractured bones, aging alcohol-associated myopathy, a discomfort and weakening in muscles caused by heavy drinking over time

malnutrition

spinal cord or peripheral nerve damage

stroke long-term corticosteroid treatment

NUTRIENTS NEEDED FOR DIABETICS AND MUSCLE ATROPHY PATIENT

High vitamin D
Low fat
Low salt (sodium)
Low carbohydrate
Moderate protein
Adequate fibre
High calcium
Anti-inflammatory and oxidative rich diet

DAY ONE:

BREAKFAST;
2 cups of whole millet pap
2 cups of beans pudding (moimoi)
2 tablespoon crayfish
2 tablespoon olive oil

MID BREAKFAST

1 medium cucumber

LUNCH

1½ cups boiled beans
½ cup rice
1 cup mixed vegetables salad (cabbage, tomatoes, lettuce)
1 oz fish (sardine, herring, salmon)
2 spoon olive oil
1 cup tomatoes source (tomatoes, onions, pepper)

MID LUNCH

2 cups skim yoghurt
DINNER {tuwon acha and okra fish soup}

1½ cups acha swallow (tuwon acha)
½ cup okra, 1 tablespoon olive oil, tea spoon locust beans (daddawa)
1 teaspoon onions paste, ½ tablespoon pepper
½ teaspoon garlic, ¼ teaspoon ginger

BED TIME
1½ cups moringa tea

Chapter 2

DAY TWO:

BREAKFAST {whole wheat bread and tea}

4 slice of whole wheat bread
1 cup skim milk

12 cups mixed vegetables (cabbage, cucumber and lettuce)
3 eggs white (boiled hard).

MID BREAKFAST

2 medium size garden eggs
½ cup unsalted roasted groundnut
LUNCH {sweet potatoes and kuka soup}

½ cup sweet potatoes swallow
2 tablespoon baobabs (kuka)
1 tablespoon crayfish
2 tablespoon olive oil
1 tablespoon pepper, 2 tablespoon onions
3 oz lean meat
1 teaspoon daddawa
MID LUNCH

1 big size pear (avocado)
DINNER {sorghum porridge}

2 cups sorghum
2 cups Amaranthus (alaiyaho)

1 cup pumpkin leaves
1 tablespoon daddawa
1 teaspoon pepper, ½ teaspoon garlic, ½ teaspoon ginger
3 oz chicken tights (skinless)

BED TIME

1 cup of skim yoghurt

DAY THREE:

BREAKFAST {boiled unripe plantain with egg source}

2 medium unripe boiled plantain
1 cup tomatoes paste and 1 cup onions paste
2 eggs
1 teaspoon pepper
2 tablespoon olive oil
2 cups of lemon grass tea and ½ teaspoon garlic

MID BREAKFAST

1 cup roasted Bambara nut
LUNCH {amala and jute soup with chicken
breast sauce}

½ cup of yam amala
½ cup tomatoes sauce
1 tablespoon daddawa
2 tablespoon olive oil
½ tablespoon crayfish
3 oz skinless chicken breast

MID LUNCH

1 cup skim yoghurt
DINNER {brown rice and green leafy
vegetables soup}

1 ½ cups brown rice
2 cups green leafy vegetable soup {pumpkin
leave (ugu), amaranthus (alaiyaho)}
3 oz fish
½ cup tomatoes, 1 cup onions, 1 teaspoon
pepper

3 tablespoon olive oil

BED TIME:

1 cup of sugar free soya milk

Chapter 3

DAY FOUR:

BREAKFAST   {finger   millet   pap   and moimoi}

2 cups of finger millet pap
2 cups Bambara nut moimoi
½ tomatoes paste, 1 cup onions
1 teaspoon pepper
2 tablespoon olive oil
MID BREAKFAST {cucumber and carrot smoothie}

1 cup cucumber and ½ cup carrot

LUNCH {rice and beans}

2 cups beans
1 cup rice
1 cup tomatoes paste, 1 cup onions
1 teaspoon pepper
½ cup bell pepper (tattasai)
1 tablespoon crayfish
2 boiled eggs

MID LUNCH

1 cup cabbage, ½ cup fresh sliced tomatoes
½ cup carrots
1 teaspoon lemon juice, 1 cup lettuce
DINNER {chicken pepper soup}

8 oz fresh chicken skinless
1 cup bell pepper [tattasai], 1 teaspoon
pepper
½ teaspoon garlic, ½ teaspoon ginger
1 teaspoon mint leave

BEDTIME

2 cups green tea

DAY FIVE:

BREAKFAST {bread sandwich and green tea}

 1 cup skim milk
1 tablespoon green tea
1 cup vegetable (cucumber, cabbage and tomatoes) {all slide}
3 eggs white

MID BREAKFAST { 1 medium avocado}

2 cups of orange juice

LUNCH {acha porridge and fish}

2 cups acha
2 cups pumpkin leaves
1 cup water leaves
¼ bitter leave

3 tablespoons olive oil
1 tablespoon crayfish
3 oz fish [sardine]
1 teaspoon daddawa
½ cup bell pepper
1 cup onions
½ teaspoon garlic, ½ teaspoon ginger

MID LUNCH

2 medium size carrot

DINNER {chicken pepper soup}

8 oz fresh chicken skinless
1 cup bell pepper [tattasai], 1 teaspoon pepper
½ teaspoon garlic
½ teaspoon ginger
1 teaspoon mint leave

BED TIME {moringa salad}

2 cups cooked moringa

½ cup sliced tomatoes
½ cup bell pepper
½ cup groundnut flake [garin kulikuli]

Chapter 4

DAY SIX:

BREAKFAST {boiled cocoyam and vegetable, fish sauce}

5 medium cocoyam [boiled]
1 cup tomatoes paste, 1 cup onions, ½ cup sliced bell pepper, 1 teaspoon pepper
½ teaspoon garlic
3 teaspoon olive oil
1 cup ugu
2oz fish

MID BREAKFAST

2 small apples and roasted groundnut

LUNCH

1 ½ cup sorghum tuwo
1 cup kuka soup
3 oz chicken breast [skinless]
1 teaspoon daddawa
2 tablespoon kuka powder
1 teaspoon of both ginger and garlic
2 tablespoon olive oil

MID LUNCH

2 cups of coconut milk
DINNER {fresh sardine pepper soup}

6 oz sardine fish
1 cup sliced bell pepper
1 teaspoon pepper, 1 cup sliced onion
½ tea spoon for both ginger and garlic
½ tea spoon daddawa

BED TIME

1 cup green tea

DAY SEVEN:

BREAKFAST {enrich pap and moimoi}

2 cups enrich pap
2 cups moimoi
1 tablespoon crayfish
½ cup tomatoes paste, ½ cup onions paste,
1 teaspoon pepper

MID BREAKFAST

1 cup skim yoghurt

LUNCH {unripe plantain amala with vegetable soup}

2 cups unripe plantain mould of amala
1 cup ogbono
¼ cup bitter leave
1 tablespoon crayfish

1 teaspoon pepper, 1 teaspoon daddawa, ¼
cup onion paste
3 oz skinless chicken thigh
2 tablespoon olive oil
1 oz dried roasted sardine fish

MID LUNCH {millet fura and skim milk}

½ cup fura and 1 cup skim milk

DINNER {beans porridge}

1 ½ cups beans
1 cup spinach
2 tablespoon olive oil
½ cup tomatoes, ½ cup onions, 1 teaspoon
pepper, 2 teaspoon bell pepper
1 tablespoon daddawa
½ teaspoon garlic

BED TIME

1 medium cucumber

NOTE: Improve physical activity level by walking twice daily for 30 to 1 hour. Swing the afflicted limbs aerobically for 10 minutes each day. Avoid sugary foods and beverages such as juices and junk food like cakes, doughnuts, biscuits, pizza, etc. Eliminate full, fatty, and sugary milk and milk products, as well as saturated and trans fats like butter and margarine. Avoid eating fatty meats, and take the skin off of birds before eating. Go for unsaturated fats like omega-3 fatty acids from fish and oils from plants like olive, avocado, soybean, and sesame. Increase your diet of dark green leafy vegetables, such as pumpkin, bitter, water, baobab, and moringa leaves. Snacks that include fruits and vegetables, such as cucumbers, lettuce, carrots, tomatoes, cabbage, broccoli, and garden eggs. Consume fruit whole rather than juice, such as oranges, avocados, pears, strawberries, and cherries. Drink herbal teas with dumba fruits (goruba), turmeric, lemongrass, mint leaves, ginger, garlic, and cloves. Choose cereals to acquire the recommended amount of fibre for bowel control and sustaining gastrointestinal tract (GIT) health. Eat legumes including beans, Bambara nuts, lentils, green beans, and peas since they are excellent sources of plant protein. Eat regularly and have at least 8 glasses of water every day. When you are under pressure, release yourself. Eat early in the day and go to bed right away. lower your salt intake Avoid processed and refined meals, as well as cold water and carbonated beverages like Fanta, Coke, and packaged sugary drinks. Consult a dietician to create a meal that will allow you to consume the required amount of calories.